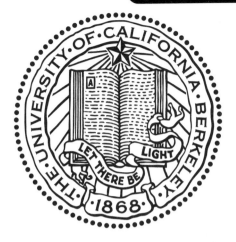

Wellness
Made Easy

365 Tips for Better Health

From the
**UNIVERSITY OF CALIFORNIA, BERKELEY
WELLNESS LETTER**

This book is based on material published in the *University of California, Berkeley Wellness Letter* in association with the School of Public Health, University of California, Berkeley.

This book is not intended to provide medical advice on personal health matters, which should be obtained directly from a physician.

A YEAR OF

WELLNESS

E very month the *University of California, Berkeley Wellness Letter* is filled with useful tips and the practical bottom line on what to do about dozens of health issues that shape your life. The advice in this book comes from recent issues of the *Wellness Letter*, a publication of the School of Public Health at the University of California at Berkeley, one of the nation's leading research and teaching institutions in this field. The *Wellness Letter* constantly reviews the latest research to give you the edge in your quest to live the best life you can.

Wellness means much more than the absence of sickness. It is a way of living that emphasizes such preventive measures as eating a healthy diet, making exercise an enjoyable part of your life, and making self-care decisions that will actively improve the quality of your life. Wellness means reducing your risk for chronic disease, preventing and treating injuries, banishing environmental and safety hazards from your home and workplace, and eliminating unnecessary trips to the doctor—but making the best use of the health-care system when you need it. This is the philosophy of the *Wellness Letter*.

The premise of wellness is that you can live a long, healthy, and active life. All you need is the desire to do so—and the right information on which to base your actions. Your subscription to the *Wellness Letter* will keep you on track.

CONTENTS

Food and Nutrition

1. Eat foods rich in vitamin C every day. An adequate intake of vitamin C may help protect against cancer and possibly other diseases. Besides oranges, the best sources of vitamin C are, in alphabetical order, asparagus, blackberries, broccoli, cabbage, cantaloupe, cauliflower, grapefruit, kale, kiwifruit, mangoes, mustard greens, peppers, raspberries, strawberries, tangerines, and tomatoes.

2. Select foods rich in carotenoids, notably beta carotene. Research shows that these substances may play a role in preventing cancer. Their orange color tells you that carrots, sweet potatoes, and cantaloupe are excellent sources of beta carotene. But so are many dark leafy greens, such as collard greens, kale, and spinach, as well as broccoli.

3. Be a semi-vegetarian. That's someone who supplements a steady diet of vegetables, whole grains, legumes, fruit, and dairy products with occasional moderate servings of beef, poultry, and fish. The potential benefits are many: a lowered risk for heart disease, cancer, and diabetes, the maintenance of a healthy weight, and fewer digestive complaints.

4. Eat tomatoes and tomato products. One four-ounce tomato supplies about one-third of your daily need of vitamin C, plus a little beta carotene, potassium, folate and other B vitamins, iron, and fiber. They are also rich in a carotenoid called lycopene, a potent antioxidant that may reduce the risk of prostate cancer and possibly some other cancers. The lycopene in cooked and processed tomatoes (sauce, paste, salsa, canned tomatoes) is more easily absorbed than that in raw tomatoes. Watermelon and pink grapefruit also contain lycopene.

5. Choose skinless turkey breast—it's just about the leanest of all meats. A three-ounce portion has less than a gram of fat and 120 calories. Plain roast turkey is your best bet: turkey cold cuts and self-basting turkeys can be quite high in fat.

6. Eat fish to help your heart. Eating fish just once or twice a week can significantly reduce the risk of heart attack. The protective value of fish comes from the type of polyunsaturated fatty acids, called omega-3s, found in its oil.

7. To cut the cholesterol you get from eggs, substitute two whites for every whole egg. Omelets can be made with whites, nonfat dry milk, and skim milk, and so can some soufflés, cakes, and muffins. Or you can substitute two whites plus one whole egg for two eggs.

8. A glass of nearly any orange juice will supply at least the daily RDA for vitamin C. Freshly squeezed juice usually has the most vitamin C, followed by frozen and canned (which retain their vitamin C for months), then by chilled cartons and unrefrigerated "drink boxes." Always check the "sell before" date. The fresher the juice, the more C.

9. Drink vegetable juice—but don't expect it to replace whole vegetables in your diet. Vegetable juices are fairly rich in vitamins and minerals but low in calories. For instance, 6 ounces typically contains about 60% of the RDA for vitamin C and nearly half the suggested daily intake of beta carotene. But vegetable juices provide little fiber (about a gram in 6 ounces). Commercial varieties tend to have lots of sodium.

10. Eat at least three servings of whole grains a day to reduce your risk of heart disease, stroke, and Type 2 diabetes. These foods include whole-grain cereals and breads, oats, and brown rice.

11. Try to avoid charred grilled meats. Cooked over high heat, fat drips onto the heating element (coals, wood, gas flames, electric coils), forming potentially cancer-causing chemicals that are deposited on the meat by the rising smoke. Such substances form whenever meat is charred; this also occurs to some extent when meat is broiled or pan-fried, especially if it's cooked until well done.

12. To reduce the risks from grilled meats, pick low-fat cuts, and trim all visible fat. Wrap meat in foil to protect it from the smoke. Don't place the meat directly over the heat source (push the coals to the sides of the grill once they are hot). Place aluminum foil or a metal pan between the meat and the coals to catch the dripping fat. And scrape off charred parts from the cooked meat.

13. Eat nuts. Many studies have now found that people who regularly eat nuts, especially walnuts or almonds, cut their risk of heart disease by as much as half. Nuts are rich in cholesterol-lowering unsaturated fats, folate and other B vitamins, heart-healthy minerals, vitamin E, arginine (an amino acid that helps relax blood vessels), fiber, and phytochemicals. The trick is to eat nuts in place of other foods. Since they have 160 to 190 calories per ounce, it is easy to gain weight if you simply add nuts to your daily fare.

14. For a juice that's high in iron, choose prune juice. One cup provides 30% of the RDA for men, 17% of that for women. Prune juice is also rich in potassium.

15. Highly nutritious foods are often low in cost. Among them are bananas, carrots, potatoes, whole-wheat flour, and dried beans—the sort of high-fiber foods that nutritionists now recommend. They also tend to come with minimal packaging—an environmental plus.

16. Keep coleslaw low-fat. It is usually more fat than it is cabbage, but you can make it low-fat. Instead of mayonnaise, try a dressing made of ½ cup plain nonfat yogurt, 3 tablespoons apple juice, and 2 tablespoons vinegar. That's enough for 1½ pounds of shredded cabbage with 2 cups of shredded carrots, 2 shredded celery stalks, ⅓ cup raisins, and 1 diced apple. Each one-cup serving has just 74 calories and almost no fat.

17. Consume enough vitamin D. Not only does it help keep bones strong, it also helps prevent falls in older people, probably by maintaining muscle function. In those over 70, a vitamin D shortfall may show up as muscle weakness, especially in the lower legs. The RDA for people over 70 is 600 IU of vitamin D a day, but 1,000 IU is a better target. Most people need to take supplements to meet this goal.

18. Read labels on muffins. A bran muffin may not even contain whole-wheat flour and may have excessive amounts of eggs, butter, and oil, as well as sugar, honey, and other sweeteners. Some have more than 20 grams of fat—as much as a Big Mac—and more than 500 calories.

19. If you're susceptible to urinary tract infections (UTIs), try cranberry juice. A study at Harvard showed that women who drank 10 ounces of cranberry juice cocktail daily significantly reduced infection rates over a six-month period. The researchers noted that cranberry juice should be used as an adjunct to medical treatment—not a substitute for it. If a UTI is serious enough to cause symptoms, it requires medical attention.

20. If you have frequent headaches, look at what you eat. Foods and beverages may play a role in some headaches, especially migraines. Most of the suspects, such as chocolate, ripe cheeses, and freshly baked yeast products, contain a naturally occurring chemical called tyramine, which may constrict or dilate blood vessels in the brain.

21. Keep bacteria out of your food. Wash your hands before starting to prepare any meal. Between steps, wash all equipment that comes in contact with food—especially raw meats—including the cutting board and countertop. Don't let cooked or refrigerated foods sit around at room temperature. Reheat foods to at least 165° F. to be sure that any harmful microorganisms are destroyed. Thaw frozen foods in the refrigerator, in cold running water, or in a microwave oven.

22. Microwaving tends to destroy fewer vitamins than conventional cooking methods. **To get the most from microwaving,** add as little water as possible to the food: a teaspoonful may be enough to prevent burning. Always cover foods while microwaving; this reduces cooking time and thus nutrient loss.

23. To get the most nutrients from your baked potato, eat the potato skin. Ounce for ounce, the skin has far more fiber, iron, potassium, and B vitamins than the flesh. The only reason to avoid the skin is if the potato has a greenish tinge. That's chlorophyll, a sign that the potato has been exposed to too much light after harvest. It's also an indication that solanine (a naturally occurring toxin) may be present in increased amounts, especially in the skin. This might cause cramps and diarrhea.

24. Try barley. It is the best source of beta glucan, a soluble fiber known to lower cholesterol. It also contains another soluble fiber called pectin, along with iron, selenium, zinc, and some B vitamins. Look for hulled barley, which retains its nutrient- and fiber-rich bran. Though its bran has been removed, pearled barley is still a good source of beta glucan.

25. High-fiber foods can help you lose a little weight. Not only are they filling and nutritious, but their fiber reduces the number of calories your body absorbs from the meal. A USDA study found that women who double their daily fiber intake from 12 to 24 grams absorb about 90 fewer calories a day from fat and protein, on average; men going from 18 to 36 grams of fiber absorb about 130 fewer calories. Nutritionists recommend at least 20 to 30 grams of fiber daily.

26. When you buy salt, choose iodized. Iodine is essential for proper thyroid functioning and for mental development. Iodine was once lacking in the American diet, especially in the Great Lakes region, where deficiency diseases such as goiter (enlarged thyroid) were once common. The introduction of iodized salt in 1922 did much to correct this. There's no need to take iodine supplements.

27. Check out broccoli. It's a powerhouse of nutrition. One cup of chopped broccoli supplies the daily requirement of vitamin C, plus beta carotene (and other carotenoids), niacin, calcium, thiamin, vitamin E, and 25% of your daily fiber needs. Not only that, but other substances in broccoli, such as sulforaphane, may also protect against cancer. All this for only 30 calories. And don't forget other cruciferous vegetables, such as cabbage, cauliflower, kale, collards, mustard greens, and Brussels sprouts.

28. Rounding out the top 10 nutrition all-stars among fruits and vegetables, along with broccoli and kale, are cantaloupe, carrots, mangoes, pumpkin, red bell peppers, spinach, strawberries, and sweet potato.

29. To get less mercury from canned tuna, choose chunk light tuna instead of albacore (solid white)—this is especially important for pregnant women and children. Albacore has, on average, about four times more mercury than chunk light, and some cans of albacore exceed the maximum mercury levels set for women of childbearing age. Light tuna, which actually is darker than albacore, comes from smaller varieties of tuna, and smaller fish tend to have less mercury.

30. To ward off strokes, eat more fruits. A large Danish study found that people who ate the most fruit had a 40% lower risk of ischemic stroke, the most common type, compared to those who ate little fruit. Citrus fruits were most protective. The likely protective elements in these foods are vitamin C and flavonoid pigments, plus an array of other antioxidants and phytochemicals.

31. Add onions and garlic to your tomato sauce. Such allium vegetables, which also include leeks and scallions, may help reduce the risk of prostate cancer in men who eat them frequently. Scallions seem to be the most protective.

32. If you take chewable vitamin C tablets because you have trouble swallowing pills, make sure you brush your teeth afterwards—or at least rinse out your mouth. A study found that 500 milligrams of chewable C can make your mouth acidic enough to start dissolving tooth enamel.

33. Here's an economical alternative to using vegetable oil spray. To cut down on the fats you use in frying foods and in greasing baking pans, just measure out half a teaspoon of oil (about 20 calories) and apply it with a paper towel or a basting brush. Or use a nonstick pan.

34. Choose dark salad greens. Romaine lettuce, for instance, not only has six times as much vitamin C and eight times as much beta carotene as iceberg lettuce, but also has more than twice as much folate, a B vitamin that is especially important for women of child-bearing age. Spinach, watercress, arugula, and chicory are other nutritious salad greens.

35. Reconsider canned corn. The heat processing used to prepare canned corn actually boosts levels of antioxidants and other healthful phytochemicals in sweet corn. Heating corn, whether on the cob or in the can, has a similar effect. The same is true of carrots and tomatoes: processing and cooking make carotenoids in them, notably beta carotene and lycopene, more readily available.

36. To reduce the calories and saturated far in your hamburger, substitute beans (such as mashed black beans) or grains (such as cooked bulgur or rice) for some of the chopped meat. The beans and grains are not just extenders: they also enhance the flavor and boost the fiber content.

37. Here's a high-fiber alternative to tomato or cream sauces on pasta: toss the cooked pasta with canned or homemade lentil or other bean soup. This is a quick version of the nutritious pasta-and-bean dishes popular in Italy. Or purée the soup before adding them to the pasta.

38. To cut down on the fat in cakes, brownies, or other baked goods, try substituting applesauce or fruit purée (such as prune, banana, or pumpkin) for an equal amount of oil, margarine, or butter in the recipe.

39. Opt for 1% or nonfat milk. Low-fat milks are not created equal. A cup of 2% milk contains 5 grams of fat and thus derives 35% of its calories from fat. A cup of 1% milk contains less than 3 grams of fat and gets 22% of its calories from fat. Whole milk contains about 3.5% fat by weight, yet this fat supplies 50% of its calories. Nonfat milk, of course, has virtually no fat, and contains just as much calcium as whole milk.

40. Eat walnuts and flaxseed. They reduce levels of C-reactive protein (a marker for inflammation associated with heart disease) in the body, as well as LDL ("bad") cholesterol and triglycerides. These foods are rich in an omega-3 fat called alpha-linolenic acid; canola oil is another source. Studies have shown that alpha-linolenic acid (as well as the other omega-3s in fish) helps reduce the risk of heart disease.

41. Add a sprinkling of poppy seeds to your green salad to give it a rich, nutty flavor, so you can use less oil. One teaspoon of poppy seeds has only 15 calories, healthy fats, and even some calcium and iron.

42. Use canned pumpkin: it's as nutritious as fresh, and that's very nutritious. A half cup has more beta carotene than a standard supplement (15,000 IU), plus a good amount of fiber, iron, and other minerals, but just 40 calories. Besides pies, you can use canned pumpkin in soups, pancakes, bread, muffins, and cookies. Or try mixing it into applesauce or plain low-fat yogurt, along with some sugar or honey.

43. Keep garlic-in-oil combinations refrigerated, whether commercial or homemade. Garlic can pick up the bacterium that causes botulism from the soil. Immersing the garlic in oil gives the spores the oxygen-free environment they need to germinate, if left at room temperature. The resulting toxin cannot be detected by taste or smell. Be equally careful with flavored oils containing herbs.

44. Try frozen fruits and vegetables as tasty, nutritious snacks. Frozen bananas, strawberries, and blueberries are delicious, and kids who won't eat cooked peas may like them straight from the freezer.

45. If you find that nonfat milk tastes watery, add a tablespoon or two of nonfat dried milk to each cup. This will help make the milk thicker and richer-tasting, and also boost the calcium and protein content.

46. Choose a roast beef sandwich instead of a hamburger at fast-food restaurants. Roast beef usually contains less saturated fat and fewer calories.

47. When shopping for whole-grain, high-fiber bread, read the label carefully. Unless the label lists whole wheat or another whole grain as the first ingredient, it's mostly refined white flour. The following terms or phrases usually mean little on a bread label: multi-grain; made with 3 natural brans; wheatberry; cracked wheat; wheat (simply white flour); stoneground (not an issue); oatmeal (usually not much); rye (ditto); sprouted wheat; unbleached (but still refined flour); or unbromated (not treated with potassium bromate—but not necessarily whole grain). Commercial rye and pumpernickel usually contain mostly white flour.

48. Compare labels on packaged deli meats. A one-ounce slice of turkey breast is almost fat-free—0.2 grams of fat in about 35 calories. Turkey bologna, on the other hand, contains 55 calories and 4 grams of fat in a one-ounce slice, which means that more than 60% its calories come from fat. One ounce of lean ham (labeled "95% fat-free" by weight) gets about one-third of its 37 calories from 1.4 grams of fat. In contrast, regular ham is 11% fat by weight, so about half the 52 calories in a one-ounce slice come from its 3 grams of fat.

49. If you like sausage but not its extremely high fat content, try one of the meatless sausage products available in health-food stores and specialty shops. These are made from vegetables, beans, grains, and aromatic herbs and spices. Besides breakfast fare, the low-fat, no-cholesterol "sausage" can be used in casseroles, pasta dishes, stuffing, or pizza. Check the label—not all vegetarian products are low in fat.

50. Gradually increase the amount of high-fiber foods you eat. Don't give up on fiber-rich grains and produce if they give you gas or cause bloating. Fiber's health benefits are many, including a reduced risk of colon cancer and constipation. Also, try a variety of fiber-rich foods until you find some that do not cause digestive problems. And drink plenty of water.

51. To remove fat from a soup, stew, gravy, or sauce, refrigerate it—the fat will rise to the top and congeal, making for easy removal. You can do this with canned stock, sauce, or broth, too. Another trick: float a paper towel on top of hot soup to absorb any remaining fat.

52. Choose colorful peppers. Ounce for ounce, green peppers have three times as much vitamin C as oranges. And red and yellow peppers have twice as much vitamin C as green ones: a whopping 170 milligrams in 3 ounces. Green peppers also supply some beta carotene, but the amount increases greatly as a pepper matures and turns red or yellow.

53. Don't rinse packaged domestic rice: it's unnecessary and it washes away some of the vitamins and minerals added to enrich it. Possible exceptions: rice purchased in bulk from open bins and some imported rices.

54. If you take calcium supplements, stick with plain old calcium carbonate, the type found in some antacids—it's by far the cheapest. All types of calcium supplements contain the amount promised on the label and all dissolve reliably in lab tests. Take calcium carbonate with food. Another good option: calcium citrate.

55. Don't take more than 500 milligrams of calcium supplements at a time. Split larger doses and take half later in the day to enhance absorption and reduce the risk of constipation.

56. When reading menus, watch out for these terms, which are giveaways to high-calorie, fatty foods: creamed, crispy, breaded, à la king, croquettes, carbonara, parmigiana, meunière, tempura, fritters, fritto, Alfredo, au gratin, au beurre, batter-dipped, bearnaise, béchamel, and hollandaise.

57. Don't assume that "natural" sodas containing fruit juice are lower in calories than regular sodas. Sometimes they actually have more calories—and only a modest amount of added nutrients. If you're trying to cut calories, stick with plain or flavored seltzers, or mix them with juice.

58. Try low-fat or fat-free tub margarines. Typically, low-fat tub margarine has only 2 grams of fat and just 20 calories per tablespoon, and nearly no heart-damaging trans fat. Standard stick margarine has 11 grams of fat and 100 calories per tablespoon, plus lots of trans fat.

59. Don't think that dry-roasted nuts are significantly lower in calories than regular roasted nuts. Because nuts are so high in fat to begin with, roasting them in oil (read: frying) hardly makes a difference. Roasted nuts absorb little oil anyway.

60. To increase the amount of iron your body absorbs from vegetarian foods, consume foods and drinks rich in vitamin C (such as orange, grapefruit, or tomato juice) with your meals.

61. Choose condiments wisely. Ketchup and prepared mustard are low-calorie, low-fat flavor boosters—just 15 calories per tablespoon—but they're high in sodium, with 150 to 180 milligrams per tablespoon. Make sodium-free mustard by mixing mustard powder with water, vinegar, or milk. Prepared horseradish has half the calories and one-tenth the sodium of mustard or ketchup.

62. Soy milk can be a good source of calcium if it is fortified with the mineral. But it usually takes about 500 milligrams of calcium in a cup of soy milk to equal the 300 milligrams in a cup of milk, since the calcium in most soy drinks is less readily absorbed than that in cow's milk.

63. Make your own low-fat, lower-calorie tortilla chips by baking fresh tortillas at 400° for 8 to 10 minutes, or until crisp. You can cut them into triangles before baking, or break them into chips afterward.

64. To preserve vitamin C, store orange juice in a tightly closed container at 40° F. or below. Whole, unpeeled oranges, however, hardly lose any vitamin C over time, since no oxygen comes in contact with the edible part. Even in a day or two of sweltering weather, an orange would lose less than 10% of its C. If you keep the fruit cool, it would dry out or rot before it lost a significant amount of vitamin C.

65. If you like the cold noodles with peanut sauce served in Chinese and Thai restaurants, make your own lower-fat version. Just mix 4 tablespoons of smooth peanut butter with the juice of a lemon, 2 teaspoons reduced-sodium soy sauce, 1 tablespoon water, and some chopped scallions. Blend and toss with cold cooked fettuccine or linguine.

66. Instead of putting a large pot of hot food directly in the refrigerator or leaving it out to cool off, place it in a deep pan of cold water (ice cubes will speed things up). Water is effective at removing heat. Once the food has cooled substantially, it can be refrigerated. One advantage of this method is that the hot food won't raise the temperature of the refrigerator.

67. Try a new fruit or vegetable every month, or every week. From the mundane to the exotic—from parsnips and artichokes to mangos and guavas—there are lots of choices, especially in farmers' markets and stores geared for various ethnic cuisines. This will help you meet the nine-a-day-minimum recommendation and will boost your intake of antioxidants and other substances that may lower the risk of cancer and heart disease.

68. Avoid fried eggplant. It soaks up oil quickly, like a sponge—more than any other vegetable, even more than French fries. Try grilling, broiling, baking, steaming, or braising it instead of frying.

69. Follow these guidelines for cooking eggs. You need not cook eggs to the hard and rubbery stage. Boiling an egg in its shell at 140° for 3½ minutes should kill virtually all bacteria. Scrambled eggs and omelets are fine if cooked just past the runny, moist stage (they should be set, but don't have to be rock hard). If you're frying eggs, "over easy" is best: fry them for about 3 minutes on one side, then about 1 minute on the other.

70. Eat sweet potatoes. Despite their sweet taste, they have about the same number of calories per ounce as white potatoes. A 3½–ounce baked sweet potato contains three times the recommended daily amount of beta carotene, half the RDA for vitamin C, and just 100 calories.

71. Avoid the typical package of ground poultry, which usually contains skin and too much fat. Look for ground turkey breast; it should be labeled 96 to 98% fat-free (by weight).

72. Try veggie burgers. They're served in many restaurants, and you'll find them in frozen, refrigerated, or mix form in the grocery store. Veggie burgers may be primarily soy and/or may contain any combination of mushrooms, onions, peppers, rice, oats, barley, bulgur (cracked wheat), rye, gluten (wheat protein), beans, spices, and egg whites. In a restaurant, ask the waiter what's in the veggie burger and how it's cooked. Some veggie burgers are almost fat-free, but some are high in fat, especially if nuts or cheese are major ingredients.

73. Eat beans and other legumes. Beans, lentils, and dried peas are all good sources of soluble fiber, which, if consumed regularly, may help lower blood cholesterol levels.

74. Cook with fresh herbs. They contain powerful antioxidant compounds, according to a USDA analysis. Herbs that scored highest by far were oregano and marjoram—just a tablespoon or two of the chopped herbs would supply significant amounts of antioxidants. Fresh herbs are more potent (in flavor and antioxidant power) than their dried counterparts, and culinary herbs in general have more antioxidant potential than medicinal ones, such as ginkgo.

75. To boost your calcium, eat sardines. When eaten with their small edible bones, three small fish (one ounce each) supply 370 milligrams of calcium, more than a cup of milk. Canned salmon, also eaten with its bones, supplies nearly as much calcium.

76. Try pink or red grapefruit. Ounce for ounce, the pink variety has more than 40 times more beta carotene than white grapefruit. And the darker the pulp, the more lycopene. This carotenoid, also plentiful in tomatoes, may help lower the risk of certain cancers.

77. Don't blindly trust those plastic pop-up timers on poultry. They work fairly well, but double-check the results. Insert a meat thermometer in the thickest part of the thigh. The temperature should reach 185°, and the leg should move easily. Juices should run clear from breast meat. Most labels also suggest that you time your bird: multiply the weight (in pounds) by 20 minutes—or more for a stuffed bird. Cook it that long even if the popper pops earlier or never pops at all.

78. Don't believe rumors about the artificial sweetener aspartame, claiming that it causes everything from multiple sclerosis, epilepsy, and brain tumors to Alzheimer's and Parkinson's disease, headaches, and blindness. Aspartame has been more intensively studied than almost any other food additive. The FDA, American Medical Association, and World Health Organization have concluded that it is safe. Aspartame's only proven danger is for people with phenylketonuria, an uncommon genetic disorder—the labels warn about this.

79. Weigh your bagel. Many fresh-baked bagels now weigh six or seven ounces and pack 500 calories or more. Plain bagels, like any plain bread, have 70 to 80 calories per ounce.

80. Choose water-pack tuna if you're trying to lose weight. It doesn't make much difference whether you choose white or light tuna, or solid or chunk. What the tuna is packed in does matter, though. Choose tuna packed in water, not vegetable oil (usually soybean oil). Even if you drain most of the added oil, what's left behind can increase the fat content of the fish three- to fivefold and the calorie count by more than 50%.

81. Limit your intake of vitamin A, since it can weaken your bones. A study found that consuming more than 6,600 IU of vitamin A from food or supplements increased the risk of fractures. The main problem is supplements: don't take a separate A pill, and check how much is in your multivitamin. And check the labels on highly fortified breakfast cereals. Beta carotene, which the body converts to vitamin A, is safe for your bones.

82. To keep dried peas and beans from causing flatulence, discard the soaking water, and don't consume the cooking water. This eliminates more than half of the indigestible carbohydrates that cause gas.

83. Don't stuff a turkey hours before cooking it. Stuff the bird only when you're ready to put it in the oven. If you refrigerate a large stuffed turkey for later cooking, the stuffing may not chill fast enough. Because any stuffing (bread or rice) is starchy, it provides an environment bacteria can thrive in. Cooking the stuffing separately is easier and safer. And don't let the bird sit around after dinner. Always remove the stuffing from the cavity and refrigerate separately.

84. Don't assume that a wine cooler is "light." It isn't: a 12-ounce bottle has more alcohol than a 12-ounce can of beer, 5-ounce glass of wine, or ounce of liquor. It also contains 150 to 300 calories.

85. It's okay to eat an egg with a blood spot. That does not indicate that an egg has been fertilized or is old. Most eggs with blood spots are removed during the grading process, but they are safe to eat.

86. Don't shy away from shellfish. Many types—notably crab, scallops, mussels, clams, and lobster—are actually slightly lower in cholesterol than chicken or beef. Even though shrimp and crayfish have about twice as much cholesterol as meat, they contain much less fat, and their fat is largely unsaturated and includes heart-healthy omega-3 fatty acids.

87. Drink the leftover milk from your breakfast cereal bowl. A significant amount of the vitamins added to fortify most cereals winds up in the milk, so it's especially nutritious.

88. Try carrot juice. A cup has as much beta carotene and vitamin C as three medium carrots. Unfortunately, it has less fiber than one carrot.

89. Don't think that fruit-only preserves are healthier. Most jams and jellies are about half fruit, half added sugar. Fruit-only preserves are usually sweetened with fruit juice concentrate, which contains fructose, a sugar with as many calories as table sugar (sucrose) and minimal nutritional differences.

90. Cook in cast-iron pots to increase the iron in foods cooked in them. The more acidic the ingredients (such as tomatoes) and the longer you cook them, the more iron ends up in the finished dish.

91. It's safe to refrigerate meat or poultry in store wrapping. Actually, by not rewrapping it you may reduce the health risks, since every time you handle raw meat you increase the chance of bacterial contamination.

92. Reconsider olives. They are high in fat, but the fat is mostly monounsaturated and thus heart-healthy. An ounce of pitted olives (about four "jumbo") averages only 30 calories and 3 grams of fat. Olives also supply some calcium, fiber, vitamin E, and healthful phytochemicals, such as phenols and lignans. The main drawback is sodium, about 200 milligrams per ounce—but you can rinse off some of this.

93. Look for lean cuts of pork. Many cuts are about one-third leaner than they were 20 years ago. The leanest is pork tenderloin, which has just 4 grams of fat and 135 calories in a well-trimmed 3-ounce cooked serving.

94. Eat that parsley. Fresh parsley contains relatively high amounts of beta carotene and vitamin C. But you have to eat about seven sprigs of it to get 10% of the RDA for these nutrients, so try parsley as a salad green, not just as a garnish.

95. Marinate meat only in the refrigerator. Don't put cooked meat or poultry back into an uncooked marinade, and don't serve the used marinade as a table sauce unless you heat it to a boil for at least one minute. The used marinade may have been contaminated by bacteria from the raw meat.

96. Skip the bacon and cheese. A bacon cheeseburger averages 250 more calories than a plain hamburger—plus a good deal more saturated fat and cholesterol.

97. When shopping for onions, look for stronger-tasting varieties. The strong taste and smell come from antioxidant compounds called polyphenols, which may reduce the risk of cancer and other diseases. Western Yellow, New York Bold, and Northern Red onions are highest in polyphenols. Shallots, though milder in flavor, also rank high.

98. Steam instead of boiling. Vegetables lose considerably less of their mineral content when steamed than when boiled.

99. When you eat yogurt or cottage cheese, don't discard the whey—the watery part that separates out and sits on top. It contains B vitamins and minerals but almost no fat. Stir the whey back into the yogurt or cheese.

100. Watch out for Japanese ramen (wheat noodles), packaged as an instant-soup "lunch-in-a-mug." They are very high in fat because they are usually dried by deep-frying in lard or palm oil. Another drawback is the high sodium content of the accompanying seasoning packet.

101. Remove the skin from chicken: this can cut the fat content by three-quarters and the calories by half. Choose the breast instead of the thigh: skinless dark meat has twice as much fat as skinless light meat.

102. Cultivate a taste for buttermilk. It actually contains no butter and usually has very little fat: most buttermilk today is made from nonfat or low-fat (1%) milk. Not just a refreshing beverage, buttermilk is also useful in cooking.

103. Handle ground meats carefully. They are more perishable—and also more likely to cause food poisoning—than other meats. Once ground, the meat has a larger surface area than whole cuts, making it an easier target for bacteria.

104. When your mouth is "on fire" from hot pepper, one way to cool it off is to drink milk (a spoonful of yogurt will also help). Hot pepper's burning component is capsaicin, which binds to your taste buds. Casein, the principal protein in milk, helps wipe away the fiery compound.

105. Speed up the ripening of most fruits by keeping them in a paper bag for a few days: this traps the ethylene gas produced by the fruit. Apples give off lots of ethylene, so you can speed the ripening of other fruits by placing half an apple in the bag with them; the apple, however, will turn mushy.

106. Try evaporated nonfat milk as a low-fat, low-calorie substitute in recipes calling for cream. A half-cup of cream has 400 calories, almost all from fat, while evaporated skim milk has about 100 and only a trace of fat.

107. When preparing lean beef, reduce normal cooking time by 20%, since it cooks faster and becomes tough when overcooked. Don't be fooled by the redness: lean pieces cooked to a medium degree may still look rare.

108. It's safe to refreeze most raw meat, provided it is handled properly and refrozen within a day of thawing. However, refreezing may adversely affect the flavor and texture of the meat.

109. Make sure your frozen yogurt is made from low-fat or nonfat milk. Brands made from whole milk (or those containing added fat) can contain as many calories and as much fat as ice cream.

110. Many fruit-containing cereals actually have little fruit in them. For a premium price, some of them have only an ounce or two of fruit in the entire box. Add your own dried fruit—or, even better, fresh fruit.

111. Don't count spinach pasta in your 9-a-day quota for fruits and vegetables. It contains little spinach—the equivalent of less than a tablespoon per cup of cooked pasta. Similarly, pasta made with other vegetable purées contains only enough for visual appeal and a hint of flavor.

112. Beware of croissants. They may seem light and airy, but they contain 12 times as much fat and 50% more calories than English muffins of the same weight—and that's *before* they're buttered.

113. Cut fruits and vegetables in thick slices or chunks to minimize vitamin losses due to exposure to air. Ideally, slicing should be done close to serving time.

114. Get extra calcium from veggies. Some contain large amounts of calcium. A cup of cooked collard greens supplies nearly half the daily RDA for calcium, and a medium spear of broccoli about one-quarter the RDA.

115. Alcohol: some good news. Heavy drinking damages brain cells, but a drink or two a day may help maintain brain function and reduce the risk of Alzheimer's and other forms of dementia, according to several recent studies. But don't start drinking because of potential health benefits.

116. And some bad news about alcohol: If you're over 65, you probably can't hold your alcohol as well as you used to. Older people get a higher blood alcohol concentration than younger people after consuming a given amount of alcohol, and are more affected by it. Alcohol is doubly risky for hip fractures, too: not only does excessive drinking increase the risk of falls in older people, but it also decreases bone density. Alcohol can also interfere with many medications older people take, as well as increase age-related driving risks.

117. You don't have to avoid all red meat. Pick lean cuts, trim visible fat, and eat small portions. Some of the leanest cuts of beef are select-grade round tip, eye of round, top round, top loin, tenderloin, and sirloin. A well-trimmed

3-ounce serving (after cooking) has less than 180 calories and 8 grams of fat—less than in skinless dark-meat chicken.

118. Check serving sizes on food labels. Some relatively small packages claim to contain more than one serving, so you have to multiply the nutrition numbers if you're planning to eat the whole thing. A 20-ounce bottle of Coke, for instance, says 100 calories, but that's for 8 ounces (the bottle of soda actually has 250 calories). Similarly, the label on a muffin, frozen entrée, or even a small bag of chips may say two or three servings.

119. To cut down on salt, try adding a few drops of lemon juice to foods. This not only perks up flavor, but also gives even a little salt more bounce. Just why a sour taste should work as an enhancer of (or substitute for) a salty one has never been explained.

120. You would have to eat two quarts of plain popcorn to get the calories in 20 potato chips. Eight ounces of potato chips contain as much fat and sodium as most people should eat in an entire day. By substituting one cup of plain, unbuttered popcorn for a one-ounce bag of potato chips, you save 135 calories and 10 grams of fat. Plain popcorn is virtually fat-free.

121. If you live or work with a smoker who won't or can't quit, eat more foods rich in vitamin C. Cigarette smoke is a major source of free radicals, which can damage cells; vitamin C and other antioxidants help inactivate these compounds, and are "used up" in the process. Passive smokers use up extra vitamin C and thus have low blood levels of this vitamin.

122. To keep vegetables fresh and nutritious, wrap them in paper towels and store them in unsealed plastic bags in the refrigerator. There are also specially designed bags for produce that allow excess moisture to escape. Don't wash veggies before storing—that only adds moisture and thus hastens spoilage.

123. Like all plain breads, pita (or pocket) bread has only 70 to 80 calories per ounce and almost no fat. Whole-wheat pita, like whole-wheat bread, is more nutritious than that made from refined wheat. Pita's main advantage is its small serving size: a typical 7-inch pita weighs only 2 ounces and has only 150 calories, versus 4 ounces or more and at least 300 calories in the average long sandwich roll or bagel.

124. Drink tea. It contains enough fluoride to help prevent tooth decay, and is also rich in substances called polyphenols, which act as antioxidants and thus may help protect against cancer.

125. Tea drinking may also help strengthen bones. Besides the fluoride, flavonoids and other compounds in tea may be good for bones. Some people still worry that tea could weaken bones because of its caffeine, but several studies have now shown this is not the case.

126. Observe the three-quarter plate rule: That's how much of the food on your dinner plate should be grains, vegetables, legumes, and fruit, leaving just one-quarter for meat, chicken, or fish. This will help you get a good mix of nutrients, control portion sizes, and cut down on fat.

127. Snack on dried fruits, but weigh the advantages and disadvantages. Because drying the fruit reduces water, it greatly concentrates the minerals (iron, copper, and potassium), beta carotene, and fiber. But it also concentrates the sugar and thus the calories; the sugar, combined with the sticky texture, makes dried fruit bad for teeth. In addition, the drying destroys most of the vitamin C and any heat-sensitive phytochemicals. About 1% of Americans, primarily asthmatics, are sensitive to the sulfites that are often added to dried fruits to preserve their color.

128. Eat kiwifruit. Ounce for ounce, it has more vitamin C than an orange and more potassium than a banana. It also supplies some folate, vitamin E, and lutein (a carotenoid that may help keep eyes healthy). This furry fruit is rich in fiber.

129. If you have a tough cut of meat, you can tenderize it with a kiwifruit. An enzyme, called actinidin, in the fruit does the trick. Just cut the kiwi in half and rub it over beef, poultry, or pork about 30 minutes before cooking. Or purée the fruit and use it as a marinade. The meat won't take on the kiwi's distinct flavor. Raw papayas contain a similar tenderizing enzyme called papain (used in commercial meat tenderizers).

130. Cottage cheese is salty (about 450 milligrams of sodium in half a cup), but the low-salt varieties don't taste very good. **As a compromise, buy low-salt cottage cheese and add one-quarter teaspoon of salt** to the 16-ounce tub. That will cut the standard sodium content by more than half. Or mix equal amounts of regular and low-salt cottage cheese.

131. You'd have to eat two cups of cottage cheese to get the calcium in a cup of yogurt or milk. Cottage cheese retains only 30 to 50% of the calcium of the milk it is made from. A cup has 100 to 200 milligrams of calcium (and dry curd has only half as much). A cup of milk has 300 milligrams; a cup of yogurt, 300 to 400 milligrams.

132. If you're trying to cut back on meats, think of a baked potato as a dinner main dish. Opened and slightly mashed with a fork, a potato can be topped with lima beans, corn, and salsa; broccoli, zucchini, mushrooms, and tomatoes can also be cooked together for a tasty filling. A small amount of Parmesan or other grated cheese will add flavor.

133. Discard most moldy fruit. Fruit molds are generally not toxic (the most toxic molds tend to grow on grains). Small fruits, such as grapes or berries, should certainly be thrown out if moldy. Cutting mold out of an apple, pear, tomato, or cucumber and then eating the fruit is usually okay. But the visible mold may not be all the mold there is—its rootlike system may penetrate the fruit—so it's important to cut widely around the mold.

134. The "imitation crab meat" used increasingly in seafood salads and salad bars is a good food, rich in high-quality protein, and with 75% less cholesterol than most shellfish. But if you're looking for heart-healthy omega-3 fats, it's a poor choice. Since it has very little fat, it has virtually no omega-3s. And it is often high in sodium.

135. If you buy bottled spaghetti sauce, check the fat and sodium content listed on the label. While most tomato-based varieties have 2 to 4 grams of fat per cup, some have 9 to 12 grams, plus more than 1,000 milligrams of sodium. The real whoppers, though, are the refrigerated sauces. Some of these cheese-based, pesto, or Alfredo sauces have half-a-day's to an entire day's worth of fat in just one serving.

136. It's safe to eat the dark "vein" running down the back of shrimp. It is actually a tiny intestinal tube. In large shrimp, it can be a little gritty, and most cooks prefer to remove it. But if the shrimp have been cooked, eating the vein won't harm you. In fact, some Southern shrimp eaters believe it actually enhances flavor.

137. Never give honey to children less than a year old. About 10% of honey contains dormant *Clostridium botulinum* spores, which can cause botulism in infants. Infant botulism is the most common form of botulism in this country, with honey the cause in approximately one-third of all cases. Honey is safe for older children, however.

138. To reduce the risk of prostate cancer, eat fish, especially fatty fish. In a Harvard study, men who ate the most fish were least likely to develop advanced prostate cancer. Fish oil supplements did not decrease the risk.

139. Don't assume that light beers are "light" in alcohol: most brands contain nearly as much alcohol as regular beer. The "light" in beer refers to calories, which must be reduced at least 25%. Light beers average about 100 in 12 ounces, versus 140 to 200 in regular beers. The lower calorie content comes from a reduction in carbohydrates, not alcohol. To avoid alcohol, try non-alcoholic beers, which contain just a trace—and, thanks to the lack of alcohol, only 50 to 95 calories per can. There's very little difference between most "low-carb" and "light" beers.

140. Even if an egg has been removed from its shell, it can still explode during or after microwaving if the yolk is left intact. The yolk's outer membrane acts like the shell: after microwaving, the yolk is very hot and under pressure, and when pierced it can explode in a person's face and cause serious burns. **Always pierce the yolk before microwaving**—or scramble the egg.

141. Pack raw meat and poultry separately from fruits and vegetables at the market. That way the meats' juices (which may contain disease-causing bacteria) won't drip on the produce. Such contamination can cause serious food poisoning if you don't wash the produce well before eating it raw.

142. To get more juice out of a lemon, orange, grapefruit, or lime, roll it on a counter or between your hands before cutting it. Microwaving also makes it easier to juice citrus fruit: microwave one fruit (taken from the refrigerator) on high for 30 to 45 seconds; two fruits, for 60 seconds.

143. For a potato chip taste–alike: Preheat your oven to 400° F., wash one large baking potato, and cut it into thin slices. Lightly coat a baking sheet with oil (you can use a spray), and arrange the slices in a single layer; brush or spray very lightly with oil, and sprinkle with paprika. Bake for 30 minutes, turning once. The slices should be crisp and brown.

144. If you like wine but want to avoid the alcohol, try nonalcoholic wines, which contain less than 0.5% alcohol. Removing the alcohol eliminates many "empty" calories, so nonalcoholic wines have less than one-third the calories of regular wine—about 20 to 30 in 5 ounces, versus the usual 100. Grape juice is another option, though it is high in calories. Like nonalcoholic wines, it contains some of the heart-healthy compounds found in wine, but lacks the heart benefits that come from the alcohol itself.

145. Watch out for chicken nuggets at fast–food restaurants. They are not a healthier choice than the burgers. Nuggets are among the fastest–growing foods in the American diet, especially among kids. Made from finely ground dark and light meat, as well as skin, they also contain lots of breading, fillers, and added fats, including artery-damaging trans fats from partially hydrogenated oils. Frozen nuggets sold in supermarkets can be just as bad.

146. If you're trying to lower your blood cholesterol, don't drink lots of unfiltered European–style coffee, such as that made in a French press (a carafe with a plunger). Large amounts of such coffee can boost cholesterol levels by 6 to 10%. The culprits are substances called diterpenes, found in oil droplets floating in the coffee as well as in the sediment. Espresso or Turkish/Greek coffee has a similar, though smaller, effect on blood cholesterol. Drip coffee (made with a paper filter) and percolated coffee contain only negligible amounts of diterpenes and thus are no problem.

147. To test how much fat is in a cracker, rub it with a paper napkin. If it leaves a grease mark, there's lots of fat in it. Even if the fat in the cracker comes from highly unsaturated vegetable oil, you don't need extra fat.

148. Beware of claims made for locally prepared foods labeled "diet," "light," or "low–calorie." Surveys show that such foods (muffins, ice cream, cookies, etc.) often weigh more and have much more fat and calories than the label says. Lax enforcement at the local level allows many food makers to get away with wild claims and boldly understated data.

149. Choose Canadian bacon instead of regular bacon to save on calories and fat. Grilled Canadian bacon, which is more like ham, has about 50 calories and 2 grams of fat per ounce (one thick slice). Regular bacon has about 165 calories and 14 grams of fat per ounce (four slices). They are equally high in sodium, however, with about 450 milligrams per ounce.

150. Don't overlook canned vegetables and fruits, which retain most vitamins and minerals. The heating process of commercial canning partially destroys certain vitamins, but some nutrient loss is inevitable whenever a food is prepared. "Fresh" produce is not necessarily more nutritious, since much of it is harvested before it is ripe, trucked thousands of miles, and stored for long periods—in which case nutrient losses can be great. Canned beans, pumpkin, corn, pineapple, spinach, and beets, to name a few, are actually quite nutritious. But watch out for added sodium.

151. Most frozen fruit-juice pops, sorbets, and ices are only very distantly related to fresh fruits or their juices. They're more like frozen sweetened water. They contain little of the fruit's vitamins (unless they are vitamin-fortified), but also little or no fat. **For a more nutritious fruity dessert,** freeze your own juice in an ice-pop mold or ice-cube tray. Or freeze canned fruit and then purée it.

152. Drain the sauce from stir-fried takeout Chinese food, since that's where a lot of the fat lurks. Or simply leave behind the last half-inch of sauce-drenched food in the container. Better yet, order steamed dishes and ask for other low-fat preparations. And share your dishes, or take most home leftovers. Entrees are usually huge—often a pound and a half each or more, enough for four "sensible" portions.

153. Forget the old rule about eating raw shellfish only during "R" months (September to April). That rule may reduce the risk of food poisoning, but certainly doesn't eliminate it. About 5 to 10% of all raw shellfish are contaminated by vibrio bacteria. People with chronic diseases or impaired immunity face a high risk of potentially fatal vibrio-related illness. Even shellfish "certified clean" is risky, since there's no way to detect many viruses and bacteria in fishing waters. To be safe, eat only thoroughly cooked shellfish (140°).

154. Always cut a hard-shell winter squash in half before microwaving. A whole squash cooked in the microwave can explode and cause serious burns. Piercing the shell with a fork before cooking may not be adequate to vent the confined steam pressure.

155. If you're grilling chicken, marinate it first—and not just for good taste. One study showed that a chicken breast marinated in olive oil, cider vinegar, brown sugar, lemon juice, garlic, mustard, and salt produced fewer heterocyclic amines than unmarinated chicken when grilled on a propane grill for 30 minutes. These substances, produced when meats are cooked at high temperatures, promote cancer. Marinating reduced some of them by 99%. If you want to consume the remaining marinade, be sure to boil it before serving.

156. Use a blender. Food processors have overshadowed blenders in recent years, but there are some things blenders do better. They purée and liquefy foods to a smoothness few processors can match. So dust off your blender to make healthy shakes and drinks. You can combine nearly any fruits with skim milk and/or nonfat yogurt to make smoothies. Try frozen ingredients, such as bananas or orange juice. You can also make vegetable "cocktails," flavorful dips, quick sauces, velvety soups, and low-fat sandwich spreads.

157. Try "melted" berries. Fresh or frozen whole strawberries or blueberries make a delicious pancake topping (replacing syrup and butter) if you "melt" them: put them in a saucepan with a little sugar, mash slightly, add a small amount of water if necessary and heat just until the sugar dissolves in the juice.

158. Use a meat thermometer not only for turkeys and roasts, but also for casseroles, egg dishes, ground meats, even leftovers. This is an especially good idea if you're in frail health. Nearly one-third of all cases of food poisoning at home are caused by inadequate cooking, according to the USDA. There are easy-to-use models that give an instant reading when inserted in food.

159. If you're a woman capable of becoming pregnant, you should consume 400 micrograms of folic acid from a supplement or fortified breakfast cereal. This B vitamin is known to reduce the risk of certain birth defects by at least 50% when consumed before conception and during early pregnancy.

160. Here are some shopping tips for crackers. Choose whole grains: whole wheat or whole rye should be the only flour, or at least the first ingredient (don't be fooled by "hearty wheat," "stoned wheat," or "multigrain" crackers, which are made from refined wheat flour). Look for at least 3 grams of fiber and less than 4 grams of fat per ounce. The fat usually comes from hydrogenated oil, with its artery-clogging trans fat.

161. Don't believe the claims made for sea salt, a favorite at health-food stores and gourmet shops. It has no nutritional advantages over regular salt. It is coarser, so it may be a little less salty per teaspoon—but if you season by taste, you'll just use more of it. By the time sea salt is cleaned and processed for the table, it's virtually identical to regular salt, though much more expensive.

162. To make caffè latte quickly and easily, use a "frother," a stove-top or microwave pot with a plunger-like top that aerates warmed milk (even nonfat milk) into a thick froth. This is a good way to increase your milk intake.

163. Choose bright and dark-colored fruits and vegetables. The color is generally a sign of extra nutrients. For instance, buy red grapes instead of green, romaine or watercress rather than iceberg lettuce, red cabbage instead of green, and dark orange carrots over pale ones.

164. Always ask your doctor or pharmacist whether medicine should be taken with food or on an empty stomach. This can affect the drug's absorption. Some drugs (prescription or over-the-counter) interfere with nutrient absorption, so if you take vitamin/mineral supplements, ask if it's okay to take them at the same time as your medicine.

165. Lead can leach out of lead crystal, especially if acidic beverages sit in it for a long period. **So don't store wine or spirits in a lead crystal decanter.** Use the decanter only for serving—pour the beverage into it shortly before you plan to use it, and then return it to its original bottle. Similarly, don't store vinegar-based dressings in lead crystal cruets. Don't worry about drinking from a lead crystal goblet—only tiny amounts of lead would be released during the short time that the wine is in the glass.

166. Try yogurt cheese as a tasty substitute for cream cheese or sour cream. It's thick, spreadable, tangy, and fat-free if you make it from nonfat yogurt. To make it, place a fine-meshed strainer or colander over a bowl and line it with one or more coffee filters, a double thickness of cheesecloth, or three layers of paper towel. Add plain or flavored yogurt (one containing no fruit, jam, or gelatin) and refrigerate overnight or longer. The longer it drains, the thicker the cheese will be. Yogurt cheese has only 20 calories per ounce. A pint of yogurt yields a cup of cheese.

167. To cut calories, start your meals with a low-fat salad. One study found that people who ate three cups of low-fat salad before lunch ended up eating 12% fewer calories at the entire meal than those skipping the salad. The key is to avoid high-fat dressings and cheese. More good news: a three-cup salad will provide at least three of the nine servings of produce you should eat daily.

168. Check the label on anything called "drink," "beverage," "punch," "juice blend," "-ade," or "juice cocktail." It is likely to contain little fruit juice—but a lot of water and sugar (generally corn syrup). Thus your "tropical punch" may contain only 10% juice, or your "cranberry juice cocktail" just 25% juice. Manufacturers must disclose the type and percentage of juices in a fruit beverage on the labels.

169. Compare "low-fat" or "low-carb" cookies and cakes carefully: Many contain nearly as many calories as conventional products.

170. If you're looking for the most nutritious yogurt, skip the fruit-flavored varieties. Most of these contain fruit jam, which is not a significant source of nutrients, but does add the equivalent of eight or nine teaspoons of sugar per cup. The jam also takes up space otherwise filled by yogurt—so jam-sweetened varieties contain less calcium, protein, and other nutrients than plain yogurt or flavors such as vanilla or lemon, which don't contain jam. The best option: add fresh fruit to plain yogurt.

171. Be careful when wiping up juices from uncooked poultry, which can contain harmful bacteria such as salmonella. You don't need a special "disinfectant" sponge or soap, just common sense. Sponges can harbor the germs and then spread them counters or dishes, even the next day. So use one sponge or dishcloth for such spills, another one for washing dishes. At the very least, wash your sponges with soap and very hot water (or use the dishwasher), and replace them often. You can use paper towels for cleaning up after handling poultry and meat.

172. Don't think that fresh pasta is more nutritious than dried. Fresh pasta often contains egg yolk and thus some cholesterol.

173. Watch what you order at the coffee bar. Plain coffee is virtually free of fat and calories. But add lots of whole milk or cream and it's a different story. Look at a mocha "grande" (16 ounces) at one national chain: almost 400 calories and 25 grams of fat. Even a merely "tall" caffè latte (12 ounces) containing whole milk has 180 calories and 10 grams of fat.

174. Catch a cantaloupe—it's the most nutritious melon. One cup (cubed) or a six-ounce slice (without skin) supplies more than the recommended daily intake of vitamin A, in the form of beta carotene. In fact, a serving of cantaloupe contains nearly 5 milligrams of beta carotene and 68 milligrams of vitamin C—nearly the daily RDA.

175. Weigh your pizza options. If, as is often the case, the slice from your local pizzeria weighs 8 ounces and is loaded with cheese and pepperoni or sausage, it probably has more than 700 calories and 40 grams (or about half-a-day's worth) of fat. Frozen pizzas, at least, have nutrition labels, so you can compare brands.

176. Bring cooking water to a boil before adding vegetables. Allowing water to heat up slowly with the vegetables in it destroys more nutrients.

177. If cooking dried beans seems like a project, try split peas or lentils. These require no soaking, so lentil or split pea soup cooks up fairly fast. Simmer the dried legumes with seasonings and cut-up vegetables until the peas or lentils are tender. You'll get lots of fiber, protein, vitamins, and minerals.

Self-Care

178. Women should know how to detect breast cancer early. Take care of yourself by performing a monthly self-exam; having an annual breast exam at your doctor's office; and having an annual mammogram starting at age 50 (women in their forties should discuss their risk factors with their doctors). Aging is the single most important risk for breast cancer.

179. All women need a regular schedule for Pap smears. You should have your first screening at age 18 or when you become sexually active, whichever occurs first. If tests are negative for three consecutive years, screening every three years is adequate.

180. Men, especially young men, should do a regular self-exam for testicular cancer. After a warm bath or shower, when the scrotal skin is relaxed, gently roll each testicle between the thumb and fingers. Feel for lumps, nodules, swelling, or a change in consistency. Be sure to examine the ropelike part called the epididymis. If you feel anything unusual, consult your doctor. Symptoms of testicular cancer include a slight enlargement of one testis and a change in its consistency. There may be no pain, but often there's a dull ache in the lower abdomen and/or groin area.

181. Get your annual flu shot—October is the ideal time. In particular, if you are over 50, have asthma, lung or heart disease, an impaired immune system, or are otherwise at high risk for serious complications from the flu, don't put off getting the shot. In fact, recent research suggests that even healthy adults under 50 (including children) can benefit dramatically and should consider getting an annual flu shot. The current vaccine is unlikely to cause side effects.

182. Though nothing cures a cold, some home remedies can help: hot drinks, especially chicken soup, can increase the flow of nasal secretions. Tea with honey temporarily relieves a sore throat. Saltwater gargles (a quarter teaspoon of salt in 8 ounces of warm water) are also helpful, as are homemade saline nose-drops (same formula as the gargle).

183. Get vaccinated against pneumonia. The shot protects against strains of pneumococcal bacteria, which are responsible for up to half of all cases of pneumonia in this country. The vaccine has few side effects, usually nothing more than a sore arm. Those over 65 should get the pneumonia shot, as well as anyone at high risk for serious or life-threatening complications from pneumonia (such as people with chronic kidney disease, diabetes, lung or heart disease, and HIV disease).

184. One of many reasons to quit smoking: a report based on the Framingham Heart Study's 26-year follow-up of over 4,000 subjects concluded that independent of other factors, "the risk of stroke increased as the number of cigarettes smoked increased." Simply by quitting, even long-term smokers can reduce this risk to the same level as nonsmokers within five years.

185. If you have low-back pain, bed rest for a day or two is generally better than a week in bed. Protracted bed rest may be counterproductive. You should begin to walk as soon as the acute pain subsides.

186. To help prevent restless leg syndrome (uncontrollable spasms in the lower leg when lying in bed), stretch or massage the affected muscles before going to sleep, and/or wear long socks to bed. The application of heat or cold compresses may help. Avoid caffeine in the evening. And don't smoke.

187. Ward off insects by using tried-and-true DEET. A study compared DEET products to seven "natural" repellants, including citronella, eucalyptus oil, soybean oil, and peppermint oil, and found that only the DEET products provide adequate, long-lasting protection. DEET has an excellent safety record when used as directed. For ordinary purposes, concentrations of 10 to 30% are adequate for adults. Use lower levels for children. Apply only on exposed skin, not under clothing; you can also apply higher concentrations directly to clothing made of cotton, wool, or nylon.

188. To increase the levels of HDL ("good") cholesterol in your blood, lose weight if you're overweight, exercise more, don't smoke, and consider a drink a day. Talk to your doctor about medication, if necessary.

189. Over-the-counter reading glasses are fine if all you need is magnification. However, it's essential to see an eye-care specialist at regular intervals for a glaucoma test and an examination, especially as you get older. Make sure that magnifying glasses are all you need.

190. Don't take antibiotics for a cold or flu. These drugs, including penicillin, are effective only against bacterial infections, such as strep throat. They can do nothing for colds or flu, which are viral infections.

191. Improve your chances of getting a good night's sleep: relax for an hour or so before getting into bed. Read, listen to music, take a warm bath. Don't take work to bed with you. Avoid strenuous exercise within a couple of hours of bedtime. Keep your bedroom quiet, dark, and cool (60° to 65° is best). Don't drink caffeinated beverages after dinner. Try to establish a regular sleep schedule.

192. There's no sure way to prevent or cure toenail fungus, but keeping your feet clean and dry may help. In addition, avoid trauma to your toes, and wear well-fitting shoes and socks. No over-the-counter product is effective for treating toenail fungus. If nail fungus is painful, see a doctor, who may prescribe a long-term antifungal drug.

193. To relieve constipation, drink more fluids and gradually increase your intake of high-fiber food. If this doesn't help within a week, see your doctor: Constipation can occasionally be a symptom of some disorder.

194. When using eyedrops, keep your eyes closed for about three minutes after putting in the drops. Otherwise your eyelids will pump out the medication.

195. To keep your teeth and gums clean and healthy, spend five minutes a day brushing and flossing. Use a fluoride toothpaste. Use a brush with soft bristles (hard bristles can damage the gums), and hold it at an angle pointed toward the junction of teeth and gums. Waxed and unwaxed floss are equally effective.

196. To reduce jet lag, use the sun to reset your body's internal clock. When flying west across several time zones, stay outdoors in direct sunlight at the end of the first day in order to help push back your bedtime and wake-up time. When flying east, go out in the sun early the next day to help you adjust to an earlier bedtime. Walk, sit, or exercise outside: wearing sunscreen won't cancel out the beneficial effect of the light.

197. Don't think that over-the-counter drugs are without risk. They can do damage if used incorrectly, and some can lead to physical dependence if overused. Read the label. Manufacturers can and do reformulate their products at higher or lower strengths, or there may be new warnings about side effects.

198. To keep a cold from spreading, wash your hands frequently. If you're around someone with a cold, avoid touching your nose and eyes. Don't share drinking and eating utensils and other objects with family members who have colds. Cover your mouth when sneezing or coughing, or sneeze into your sleeve. Dispose of used tissues promptly in a plastic-lined wastebasket or paper bag, or in any manner that makes rehandling them unnecessary.

199. Chew sugarless gum to help fight tooth decay. Gum chewing stimulates saliva flow and thus reduces harmful acidity from bacteria in the mouth. It also helps squeeze saliva into the spaces between the teeth. To get the most benefit from gum, pop a stick into your mouth within five minutes after eating and chew it for at least 15 minutes.

200. If you have hay fever, cut down on alcoholic beverages during pollen season. They cause blood vessels in the nose to swell, thereby further increasing nasal congestion.

201. Count your moles to gauge your risk of malignant melanoma, the most dangerous form of skin cancer. If you have six or more large moles, 5 millimeters or larger (about one-fifth of an inch, the size of a pencil eraser), you're at increased risk and should check your skin frequently and have a professional skin exam. The moles can be flat or raised, pigmented or flesh-colored. For hard-to-see areas like your back, ask someone else to count the moles. Any mole that changes size, texture, or color, or that itches, burns, or bleeds should be checked by a doctor.

202. To prevent heartburn at night, try elevating the head of your bed by at least six inches (wooden blocks will do the trick). This may prevent the most common cause of heartburn—gastroesophageal reflux, the backup of stomach contents into the lower esophagus, where gastric acids produce a burning sensation.

203. If you have a tooth knocked out, call your dentist right away and try to get to the office ASAP. You have a 50% chance of a successful replantation if you get to the dentist within 30 minutes. You may be advised to insert the tooth in the socket (after gently rinsing it) and bite down on it until you get to the office.

204. To be sure that you are drinking "plenty of fluids," especially when you have a cold or flu, drink enough to keep your urine clear and pale in color. If your urine is deep yellow, you may not be drinking enough.

205. Don't open time-release capsules and swallow the contents. The medicine may be absorbed into the bloodstream too quickly.

206. You should have a tetanus booster—actually a combined tetanus and diphtheria (Td) shot—every 10 years. Because immunization is so widespread, relatively few cases of tetanus occur in this country anymore. But about 70% of tetanus infections occur in people over 50, who are least likely to be adequately immunized. Tetanus is not caused just by rusty nails and the like. The disease, often fatal, can be caused by even minor wounds or scratches.

207. If you're considering taking low-dose aspirin to prevent heart attacks, talk to your doctor first. Like any medicine, aspirin is not risk-free: it can cause stomach pain, heartburn, nausea, and intestinal bleeding. Anyone taking a daily dose of aspirin needs a doctor's supervision.

208. If you're a light sleeper, try a white-noise machine. This masks irritating noise with a hum or dull roar that is less noticeable than sudden sounds. You can also use a fan or air conditioner to block out noise.

209. If your muscles are sore the day after a strenuous bout of exercise, ibuprofen or aspirin (but not acetaminophen) can provide relief. Resting the sore muscles can ease the discomfort, but "active rest" may be better: repeat the activity that caused the soreness, but at a low intensity (for instance, walk, don't run).

210. If you have insomnia, don't reach for a drink. Alcohol may help you fall asleep, but your sleep will be unsettled. After a nightcap, you may wake up in the middle of the night and not be able to get back to sleep.

211. Don't worry about the mercury in dental fillings. There's no evidence to support the claim that the mercury used as a hardener in silver dental amalgams can leach into your bloodstream and cause disease.

212. If you think you have a splinter in your finger, but aren't sure, here's an easy way to find out. In a dark room, put a small flashlight directly against the finger. You should be able to see, from the side, how deep and how large the splinter is, making removal easier.

213. If you have trouble swallowing pills, take a swallow of fluid before you put the pill in your mouth—advance lubrication helps. And put the pill or capsule as far back on your tongue as possible. Try drinking from a soda bottle or any similar bottle: by keeping your lips on the bottle as you drink, you'll set up a sucking action that makes the pill go down.

214. If you slam your finger in a door or hit your finger with a hammer, you can reduce the risk of losing the nail by immediately squeezing the fingertip and keeping pressure on it for about five minutes. This minimizes internal bleeding and swelling, which can displace the nail root from its bed. Icing can help, too.

215. To halt a calf cramp, try flexing your foot by pointing it upward. Lying down and grabbing the toes and ball of your foot and pulling them toward your knee may help. At the same time, massage the calf muscle gently to relax it fully. Walking may help, too, particularly if you put your full weight on your heels.

216. Use only a water–based lubricant (such as K–Y Jelly) on latex condoms. Oil-based products, including petroleum jelly, mineral oil, cold cream, vegetable oil, and hand lotion, cause latex to deteriorate in as little as one minute. The label should say that the lubricant is safe for latex.

217. If you're one of the many women who find women's shoes too narrow, buy your exercise shoes in the men's or boys' department. Men's shoes tend to be cut wider up front. This can make a big difference, because exercise puts so much stress on the ball of your foot and your toes.

218. If you are substantially lighter or heavier than average, ask your doctor or pharmacist about adjusting the standard doses of over-the-counter medications. For instance, if you weigh over 200 pounds, you may be told to take three aspirin. Your weight, amount of body fat, age, sex, and fitness level all affect how your body absorbs and utilizes drugs.

219. When talking to someone who is hard of hearing, lower the pitch of your voice. Hearing loss in most elderly people primarily involves high-pitched sounds. Talking loudly may be counterproductive, since it usually makes you raise the pitch of your voice along with the volume.

220. Don't take an antacid that contains aluminum if you are taking any prescription drug—first consult your doctor or other health-care provider. Labels on such antacids warn about possible drug interactions.

221. Don't try to suppress a sneeze. If you hold your breath, seal your lips, and pinch your nose while sneezing, you create enormous pressure in your nose and throat, which can force infections into your sinuses or ears.

222. If you often suffer from ear pain when flying because of changing cabin pressure, take a decongestant. The descent can be especially painful, so take the pill at least one hour before landing. Or use a decongestant spray (for your nose) before landing. Decongestants won't help in children under six, however. You can also try EarPlanes, silicone ear plugs with a filter that gradually equalizes the effects of changing pressure. They cost about $5 in drugstores and airport shops.

223. Avoid whispering if you are hoarse. Whispering is usually worse for injured vocal cords than normal speech, since in most people whispering is frictionally produced sound. It's best, when hoarse, to rest your voice as much as possible; otherwise speak in a soft, confidential tone.

224. For a painful arch: roll your foot over a can of frozen juice concentrate. Both the cold and the massage will help relieve the pain. If the can is too cold, wrap it in a washcloth. You can also use a can of tennis balls or any other can to massage the arch, but you won't get the icing effect.

225. The health benefits of birth control pills far outweigh the risks for the great majority of women. Not only do they provide safe, reliable contraception, they reduce the risk of ovarian and endometrial cancer. The risk decreases the longer the pill is used, and this benefit lasts at least 15 years after use is discontinued. Women at high risk for ovarian cancer can help protect themselves by taking the Pill.

226. Ice a headache. Apply the pack where the pain is centered on your head or upper neck as soon as possible. Reusable gel packs, kept in the freezer, are handy, comfortable, and, according to one study, provide at least some relief in as many as 70% of headache sufferers. Running cold water over your head may have a similar effect.

227. If you are over 65, ask your doctor about the doses of over-the-counter medications you take regularly. Many older people do not need—and should not take—full adult doses. Age-related changes in the liver may increase the amount of medication in the bloodstream, resulting in greater therapeutic effects, as well as potential side effects.

228. If you are allergic to dust mites and suspect that your area rugs make you sneeze and itch, place them outdoors in direct sunlight. In one study, Australian researchers placed mite-infested rugs upside-down on an outdoor concrete surface during a summer day. After four hours, no live mites or eggs survived. Airing rugs and other household items outdoors dries and warms them, a process that kills mites.

229. If you have an ingrown toenail, soak the toe in water to soften the nail, then wedge a few strands of absorbent cotton (or unwaxed dental floss) under the corner of the nail to keep it from cutting the skin. Do this several times a day, if necessary, until the nail grows out. To prevent painful ingrown toenails: when trimming the nails, always cut them straight across. And don't trim toenails too close.

230. If you are prone to ear infection and your ear begins to itch after swimming, use antiseptic eardrops—particularly if you've been swimming in a lake. You can buy these without a prescription at any drugstore. Or mix equal parts white vinegar and rubbing alcohol, and put one or two drops in each ear with a medicine dropper three times a day.

231. To reduce the risk of carpal tunnel syndrome, a painful disorder of the wrist and hand, keep your wrists straight when working with your hands. (Flexing and twisting them stresses the carpal tunnel.) If you're working at a computer keyboard, make sure your fingers are lower than your wrists; don't rest the heel of your hands on the keyboard. And avoid working in the cold, which reduces blood flow and can promote carpal tunnel syndrome.

232. If you have pinkeye or another eye infection, don't use an eye patch unless your doctor tells you to: the patch can encourage the growth of infectious organisms.

233. To save money on drugs, ask your doctor about prescribing tablets that are double your needed dosage, which you can cut in half. Many tablets come scored with a line for ease of cutting. Often a tablet that's twice as potent costs only 25 to 50% more. This won't work for all medications, and you must be careful to make sure you cut the tablet evenly in half. The best way to do this is to use a special pill cutter, which is inexpensive.

234. If you know a smoker who won't quit because of the fear of weight gain, pass on this news. Smokers usually do gain weight during the first year or two after quitting, but a Canadian study found that afterwards most female ex-smokers (but fewer men) lose all or most of the extra pounds. It also found that two years after quitting, the women were actually less likely to be obese than were smokers. As a means of staying thin, smoking is a poor bargain.

235. When buying shoes, always have your feet measured, since their size may have changed if you've gained or lost weight or started exercising more. Put your full weight on the foot as it's being measured. Most of us have one foot that's larger than the other; choose the size that fits the larger foot. Feet expand during the course of the day, so go to the shoe store midday or later, when they'll be their "true" size.

236. If vacuuming intensifies your allergies, get microfiltration bags for your vacuum cleaner. These have a two-ply design that can trap many of the smallest particles. Such filters cost more than the standard ones and may fit only certain vacuum models and brands. There are also electrostatic filters that fit over the exhaust of some vacuum models. For the most effective removal of allergens, consider buying a vacuum cleaner with a HEPA (high-efficiency particulate arresting) filter, a type of filter found in the best air purifiers.

237. Switching from cigarettes to a pipe or cigars does not eliminate risk. Cigars and pipes increase the risk of not only cancer of the mouth, but also lung cancer, since former cigarette smokers tend to inhale.

238. Don't forget your lips when applying sunscreen: the lower lip is one of the most common sites for skin cancer. You can use a clear or colored sunscreen lipstick or, for even more complete protection, zinc oxide (an opaque sun block). These products also help prevent lip chapping and blistering from the sun—and may help some people avoid the recurrence of cold sores.

239. Don't use hydrogen peroxide for cleaning wounds. It is no more effective than soap and water (still the preferred method), and may actually damage the surrounding healthy skin.

240. To prevent dry skin, limit bathing to 15 minutes a day, and favor a tepid shower over a hot bath. Excessive bathing in hot water, and the excessive use of strong soap, washes away the natural oils that help trap water in the skin. Use a very mild soap, and dilute it with water rather than lathering it directly on your skin. Apply a moisturizer immediately after bathing or showering.

241. For the greatest protection from the sun, get a sunscreen with titanium dioxide or zinc oxide. Or use a product—these are now widely available—with avobenzone (also called Parsol 1789). This protects against the widest spectrum of UVA rays. Other sunscreen ingredients absorb mostly UVB rays, which are mainly responsible for sunburn and the less deadly skin cancers. UVA rays may be more important in the development of melanoma, the most deadly skin cancer, as well as wrinkling and leathering.

242. Apply sunscreen at least 30 minutes before you go out into the sun. This allows the active ingredients to penetrate the topmost layer of skin and makes them more effective. Use a generous amount, not a little dab, and reapply frequently.

243. Call your doctor for test results—don't assume that no news is good news. One-third of doctors do not always notify patients of abnormal test results, according to one study. The most common reasons for not notifying patients were that the patient was expected to return to the office/clinic soon or that the results were trivial. Many of the doctors didn't even make a record when they did notify patients.

244. To reduce the risk of osteoarthritis, maintain a healthy weight, since obesity stresses the joints. According to a long-term study of students at the Johns Hopkins School of Medicine, young men in their twenties who are 20 pounds or more overweight nearly double their chances of developing arthritis of the knee and hip later in life.

245. Brush your teeth after sucking on hard candies. These are more likely to cause tooth decay than are sweets such as ice cream or cake, since the candies dissolve slowly and surround the teeth with sugar. By the way, raisins, which are sticky, can cause more cavities than chocolate.

246. Avoid raking leaves if you're allergic to molds. The risk of allergic reaction is less if you rake freshly fallen leaves, since it takes a day or two for molds and mildew to develop.

247. When shopping for a pain reliever or cold medication, avoid multi-ingredient drugs. They cost more and provide less of the ingredient you seek. If you have a cold, buy a simple decongestant (if you want one). If you have a headache and an upset stomach, buy a pain reliever and an antacid..

248. Drink plenty of fluids if you often have bad breath. The most common cause of short-term bad breath is a dry mouth. Brush and floss to improve your breath; if you can't, try rinsing with plain water.

249. Don't store medications in the bathroom. The high heat and dampness from the bath can speed the deterioration of drugs. Choose a cool, dry place—such as a closet shelf (a high shelf if you have kids).

250. Don't expect coffee to sober you up. Even the strongest brew will not restore your motor reflexes or your sense of judgment if you've drunk too much.

251. Stay out of tanning booths. These use high-intensity light sources emitting chiefly ultraviolet A (UVA) radiation, which deeply penetrates the skin and causes premature aging. This radiation may also damage blood vessels and even inhibit immune reactions in the skin.

252. Have your tap water tested for lead if your household includes a small child or a pregnant woman. Call your local health department or water company; it may offer free or inexpensive testing.

253. If you often encounter aggressive dogs along your exercise route, try carrying one of the following for self-defense: a dog repellent (one type is ground pepper in aerosol form), a device that emits high-frequency sound waves, a water pistol, or a pop-open umbrella.

254. If your reaction time isn't as fast as it used to be, consider defensive driving training. Most localities will remove citations for moving violations, if any, from your permanent driving record when you complete a course. Most insurance companies offer graduates a break on premiums.

255. When driving, the best position for your hands on the steering wheel is at the 9 o'clock and 3 o'clock position (not at the 10 o'clock and 2 o'clock position most of us were taught). This will give you maximum control.

256. Grandparents: don't leave medication around the house within reach of young grandchildren. Childhood poisoning often involves a grandparent's medication. Use child-resistant containers. Vitamin and mineral pills (especially iron) can also be a hazard.

257. During a thunderstorm, don't bathe or shower. If the building is struck by lightning, plumbing can conduct electricity. And don't use a phone that's attached to the base by a cord. Using a cordless phone indoors is safe, but a cell phone outdoors may attract lightning.

258. Don't drink alcohol before swimming or while boating. Anywhere from 25 to 50% of adolescents and adults who drown while swimming or die in boating accidents consumed alcohol beforehand.

259. Small children should ride in car safety seats, of course, but never in the front seat. This is especially true if the car has a passenger-side air bag. All kids under 12 should ride in the rear and always be buckled in.

260. Whether you are driving or on foot, beware of cars turning left at intersections. Though only about 15% of all vehicles at intersections turn left, 45% of auto collisions and about 30% of collisions with pedestrians involve a left-turning vehicle, according to one study.

261. Don't use hanging pest strips, since these constantly release pesticide into the air you breathe. In addition, many of them contain a known carcinogen.

262. Don't leave mouthwash within the reach of young children. Many brands of mouthwash contain more alcohol than wine and can be harmful to small children.

263. Make sure that young kids don't use more than the recommended "pea-size" amount of toothpaste and that they don't swallow it. Fluoride is crucial in protecting teeth, but the large amounts in toothpaste, if swallowed frequently, can cause mottling (fluorosis) of the enamel of permanent teeth.

264. Never mix household cleaning products. For instance, the combination of chlorine bleach with an ammonia cleanser or a dishwashing liquid gives off a toxic gas that's a severe respiratory irritant.

265. Place healthy infants less than six months old on their backs or sides at bedtime (not on their stomachs, which is what most parents believe they should do). This may reduce the risk of sudden infant death syndrome (SIDS)—also known as crib death—by as much as 50%. Never put an infant on top of fluffy bedding, pillows, or comforters.

266. Remove drawstrings from hoods and necks of children's clothing, or at least cut the strings as short as possible. Drawstrings can get caught on playground equipment, an escalator, a fence, or elsewhere.

267. Women on weight-loss diets should consume extra calcium. One study found that overweight postmenopausal women who lost weight on a diet absorbed less calcium from food and supplements than women not on a diet. Women over 50 are supposed to consume 1,200 to 1,500 milligrams of calcium a day, but this study suggested that 1,800 milligrams is a better goal for dieters.

268. Don't take any over-the-counter pain reliever for more than 10 days, unless advised by your doctor. Aspirin, ibuprofen (such as Motrin or Advil), and naproxen (such as Aleve) can cause gastrointestinal bleeding and ulcers. High doses of acetaminophen (such as Tylenol) can damage the liver. The risks are greatest in heavy drinkers and those with kidney disease.

269. If you have a manicure at a nail salon, make sure all instruments have been sterilized in a disinfection machine or hospital-grade disinfectant. This will prevent the spread of infections. Just dipping the instruments in alcohol or that ubiquitous blue dip is not enough.

270. Don't worry about swallowing pits and seeds in fruit—or even an entire apple core. Actually, this will give you extra fiber. Many seeds are both edible and nutritious. Some seeds or pits (apple, apricot, pear, cherry, and plum) contain a minute quantity of a substance called amygdalin, which releases cyanide. This is not usually a health hazard. You would have to consume 50 to 70 apricot pits to get a lethal dose of cyanide.

271. Watch for these signals of sleepiness when driving: you suddenly realize you can't recall the last few miles of highway, and you're not sure where you are; you "come to" as your car veers toward the shoulder or into another lane; you have trouble keeping your eyes open and focused; or you notice an obstacle but barely manage to brake fast enough. Pull over and rest. Consider stopping for the night if possible.

272. Don't mix driving and sleeping pills. The pill you take at night can impair your driving ability for up to 17 hours.

273. Don't walk under the influence. About half of all adult pedestrians killed in traffic accidents in recent years had been drinking, and more than a third were legally drunk.

274. If you have low-back pain and are shopping for a mattress, buy a medium-firm one, not a hard one. Conventional wisdom, along with many mattress ads, claim that firmer mattresses are better for your back. But a Spanish study of people with chronic back pain found that a mattress of medium firmness is more likely to reduce symptoms. Your mattress is a health issue, however, only if it is uncomfortable and interferes with your sleep and/or leaves you with a backache.

275. Install a carbon monoxide detector. And take these steps to keep this odorless but deadly gas out of your house: have your heating system professionally inspected and tuned up annually. Vent all fuel-burning space heaters and gas ranges to the outside. Run an exhaust fan and keep a window open slightly while you cook; make sure the stove's flame is blue (if it's yellow, call your local gas company and ask to have the burner adjusted). A pilot light that is on all the time is another source of emissions.

276. To avoid traveler's diarrhea in developing countries, take these precautions: drink only bottled or canned beverages, and be sure you're the one who breaks the seal. Or stick to hot drinks made with boiling water. Never use tap water, even for brushing your teeth. Pass up ice cubes. Don't eat anything raw. Raw fruit is okay if you peel it—don't wash it in tap water.

277. Never shake an infant or young child. Since a young child's neck muscles are weak, this can cause brain or spinal-cord damage.

278. Whether you use wood or plastic for cutting raw meat and poultry, **scrub the board well afterward with hot soapy water,** and wash the knife and your hands thoroughly as well. Cutting boards are prone to bacterial contamination from food. If the surface has fat on it, or if the plastic is deeply scarred, it's especially important to get it very clean. A plastic board has the advantage of being dishwasher-safe.

279. Don't skip your seat belt just because you have an air bag. Safety belts reduce driver fatalities by 42%; add an air bag and you gain another 6%. But the air bag alone reduces fatalities by only 18%. Moreover, the impact of an air bag can be dangerous if you aren't belted.

280. Use lead-glazed earthenware pottery only for ornamental purposes. Some pieces—especially those from Mexico, China, and many developing nations—may leach lead into foods.

281. If you have heart disease, or even if you have risk factors for it, avoid indoor settings that allow smoking. Smoke increases the risk of a heart attack by rapidly increasing the tendency of blood to clot, which can restrict flow to the heart, and by causing other adverse effects in the arteries.

282. If you skid when driving: take your foot off the brake and the accelerator, and shift into neutral. Look and steer in the direction you want the front of the car to go. As soon as the wheels grip the road again, return to driving gear and slowly accelerate.

283. If you have crowns or bridges, work hard to keep them clean. The tooth base that holds a crown can decay, and crowns and bridges can attract and hold plaque (the film in which harmful bacteria live) and thus increase your risk of periodontal disease. Floss thoroughly at least once daily and brush at least twice. Brush at the gum line with a soft brush, and aim the bristles at a 45° angle to the gum line. If you have extra space between your teeth, use an interdental brush—a tiny brush tip at the end of a handle. To clean around fixed bridges, use a floss threader to get the floss between the bottom of the bridge and your gums.

284. If you often have bad breath, gently brush your tongue when you brush your teeth. Brush the back of the tongue to remove odor-causing bacteria lodged on the surface. Consult your dentist to make sure that gum or tooth disease is not the culprit. Most people can't tell if and when they have bad breath unless someone tells them.

285. Many women still don't know that some oral contraceptives can serve as "morning-after" pills. Called emergency contraceptives, these pills can prevent an unwanted pregnancy if taken within 72 hours (the sooner, the better) after intercourse. They reduce the chance of becoming pregnant by at least 75% and have only minor side effects.

286. With herbal "remedies," it's buyer beware. There is no testing for safety or effectiveness. In addition, there's no guarantee that they are what the labels say they are, that the dosage is accurate, or that the next bottle will have the same ingredients.

287. Measure your waist to find out if you are at risk for weight–related health problems. More than 40 inches in men, and 35 inches in women, is a sign of significant abdominal obesity and increased risks, regardless of height. But those are not magic numbers: there's some evidence that risk starts to rise before those cutoff points.

288. If you grind your teeth at night, your dentist can create an individually fitted mouth guard or splint made of soft or hard acrylic. Usually worn at night, the guards redistribute the forces exerted while grinding and thus help protect teeth. They can cost $300 or more. You can try a simple athletic mouth guard, sold at sporting-goods stores for around $5. If it fits properly, it should spread the clenching pressure evenly across your mouth. It won't be as comfortable as a custom-made device and will certainly be bulkier and more visible.

289. Don't handle poison ivy roots or stems—all parts of the plant can be toxic, even if they're dead. If you're trying to rid your yard of poison ivy, kill it with an herbicide. Then, wearing gloves and heavy protective clothing, bury the dead plant. Don't burn it: that can send the toxic oil airborne. Afterwards, be careful when removing the gloves so that you don't transfer the oil to your skin. The oil, like the plant, is extremely hardy: touching an object (a shovel or shoe) that was contaminated even months earlier can cause a rash.

290. Follow this shadow rule for sun protection in the summer: If your shadow is shorter than your height, it's sunburn time. In most parts of the country, this test will show that you can still get burned between 3 p.m. and 4 p.m. The sun is closest to directly overhead—and thus strongest—about 1 p.m. (Daylight Saving Time). Protect yourself with sunscreen and clothing during the three hours before and after this peak time.

291. To boost the analgesic effect of pain relievers, take them with caffeine. One study, for instance, found that a pill containing acetaminophen (as is found in Tylenol) along with caffeine was substantially more effective against headache pain than plain acetaminophen. You don't have to buy special caffeinated pain relievers to get this effect. Taking aspirin with a caffeinated beverage such as coffee or cola increases the aspirin's effect.

292. If you have trouble falling asleep, look at the ingredients in any pain relievers you're taking—several brands of aspirin and acetaminophen contain caffeine. Two of these tablets typically contain 130 milligrams of caffeine, as much as in a cup of coffee.

293. If you often have heel pain (especially first thing in the morning) or tight Achilles tendons (located behind the ankle), try this simple calf stretch. Stand with the balls of your feet on a step or curb, and slowly dip your heels as low below the step as you can. Hold the stretch for 10 to 15 seconds. Use the handrail for balance. Repeat 10 to 20 times.

294. In case you start choking on food when no one is around to help, you should know how to do the self-administered Heimlich maneuver. Make a fist and place the thumb side against your abdomen, slightly above the navel. With the other hand, grasp the fist and press it in and upward with quick, sharp thrusts. Another method: press your abdomen (just below the ribs) forcefully against the back of a chair, table, sink, or railing. Repeat until the food is expelled.

295. Keep hard objects stored under the seat or in the glove compart-ment while you're driving. Books, pens, cups, brushes, de-icing tools, and other paraphernalia can turn into missiles if they get in the way of a deploying air bag or if you have to brake suddenly or are in a crash.

296. No sex please: If you are scheduled for a PSA (prostate-specific antigen) test, which helps screen for prostate cancer, do not ejaculate for about 48 hours beforehand. Ejaculation temporarily boosts PSA levels, which could lead to a false-positive result, further testing, and even an unnecessary biopsy.

297. Never put butter or mayonnaise on a burn. Cold water, which eases the pain as it cleanses, is the most effective first-aid treatment for a first-degree burn (defined as a burn involving only the outer skin layer). Use ice wrapped in a towel if it's not practical to immerse the burned area. Butter or mayo will trap heat, slow down healing, and increase the risk of infection. Burn ointments have similar drawbacks.

298. Don't worry about "catching" a sexually transmitted disease from a toilet seat. The intact skin has an extremely able line of defense against harmful viruses, bacteria, and other would-be intruders. As long as the skin of your thighs and buttocks is unbroken, you have virtually no chance of getting a dis-ease from a toilet seat.

299. If you often have heartburn (esophageal reflux) at night, try sleep-ing on your left side. That position will keep the acidic contents of your stom-ach below the juncture with the lower esophagus, thus reducing acid backup into the esophagus.

300. Make sure your smoke detectors are in working order. Surveys show that most home owners never test their smoke detectors and that up to half of all smoke detectors are not working because of poor maintenance. Test the bat-tery every year and replace it regularly, according to the manufacturer's instruc-tions. One good way to test the device is to use an aerosol tester (about $5 at hardware stores) that simulates smoke. Replace any smoke detector that's more than 10 years old. Reliable, battery-powered, state-of-the-art smoke detectors can cost as little as $10.

301. If your eyes are sensitive to glare when driving at night, ask an optometrist or optician to put an anti-reflective coating on your regular eyeglasses. If you don't wear prescription lenses for driving, you might get plain glasses with this coating just to keep in the car. Do not wear sunglasses for nighttime driving.

302. If your car's air conditioner makes you sneeze, the culprits are probably fungi that produce airborne mold spores and grow deep within the A/C system. To minimize this problem, keep the car windows open part way for 10 minutes after you turn on the A/C. Don't direct the vents toward your face. Use "fresh air" rather than recirculated air. If these steps don't help, have your car treated with an EPA-registered disinfectant, available at car dealers, some service stations, and auto A/C shops.

303. If you are taking medication to lower your cholesterol levels, don't think it's no longer necessary to have a healthy diet. Unlike the drug, a semi-vegetarian diet reduces the risk of heart disease in several ways. Not only does it help lower blood cholesterol, it also supplies antioxidant vitamins and certain B vitamins that may help prevent heart disease (and possibly cancer). A healthy diet will also help you lose weight.

304. When using a halogen lamp, especially a floor lamp, beware of fires. These lamps get exceedingly hot, so they can easily cause fires if they fall over or if something falls onto the bulbs. New lamps must meet stricter safety standards: for instance, they must have emergency cutoff switches and metal grates on top.

305. To prevent athlete's foot, keep your feet clean and dry, especially in hot weather. Snug, poorly ventilated shoes and damp, sweaty socks provide an ideal breeding ground for the fungus that causes athlete's foot. Daily washing with soap and water is a good idea, but be sure you dry thoroughly, particularly between the toes (you can use a hair dryer on low heat). When you can, go barefoot. Next best thing is to wear sandals. When you wear shoes, wear clean socks, too, preferably ones that "wick" away moisture. Air your shoes between wearings—don't wear the same pair day in, day out.

306. Don't use a portable heater, lantern, or stove while sleeping in enclosed areas such as a tent, camper, or other vehicle. Every year about 30 Americans die and 450 are seriously harmed by carbon monoxide poisoning from the use of such devices in tents or campers. High altitudes and alcohol consumption worsen the effects. Carbon monoxide is especially toxic for infants, pregnant women, the elderly, smokers, and those with heart disease.

307. Lick your wound. Of course it's best to wash it with water, but licking a wound is a time-honored practice that may actually help disinfect it and promote healing, according to a small English study. Researchers found that nitrites in saliva react with the skin to make nitric oxide, a chemical that can kill bacteria. Saliva also contain other substances that can help in healing. For scrapes and cuts that are hard to keep clean, try Betadine (povidone iodine).

308. If you're using sunscreen and an insect repellent containing DEET, apply extra sunscreen and reapply it often. A concentration of 30% DEET spread on top of a sunscreen with SPF 15 decreases the effectiveness of the screen by about 40%, according to one study, probably because DEET is a solvent. Combination products, containing both DEET and a sunscreen, are available, but the separate products are better because you can keep reapplying sunscreen without having to reapply the DEET.

309. Think twice before buying an iguana if you have young children in the house. These reptiles are responsible for thousands of cases of salmonella poisoning each year. Researchers believe that households where the reptiles roam about have a "veneer" of feces that contain the salmonella bacteria, which then gets on people's hands and then into food. So don't let a pet reptile wander through your house. Wash your hands, and make sure your kids wash theirs, after handling one.

Fitness

310. Be active. As many as 12% of all deaths—250,000 per year—in the U.S. may be attributed indirectly to lack of regular physical activity. Only about one in four Americans exercises enough to be considered physically active.

311. Walk to lose weight. A 200-pound person who starts walking a mile and a half a day and keeps on eating the same number of daily calories will lose, on average, 14 pounds in a year.

312. Do aerobic exercise, such as running, brisk walking, cycling, or swimming. These workouts strengthen your heart and circulatory system. Try to do this three times a week for at least 20 minutes.

313. To get the most from your aerobic exercise, figure out your target heart rate. The easy way to compute this is to subtract your age from 220—that's your maximum heart rate (MHR)—then multiply that figure by 60% and 80%. For example, if you're 40, your MHR is 220 minus 40, or 180. Then multiply 180 by 0.6 (for the low end) and by 0.8 (for the high end), which gives a range of 108 to 144. Then take your pulse while exercising. Your heart rate per minute should fall somewhere between these two numbers.

314. Don't worry that exercise will increase your appetite. Most people who work out moderately eat about the same as they would if they didn't exercise—or just slightly more. By exercising regularly you're likely to become trimmer and fitter even if your weight stays the same, since you'll be building muscle and burning body fat.

315. Exercise to improve your mood and give yourself an energy boost. Many people experience an uplift in mood after a run, a swim, or a brisk walk, and numerous studies support this salutary psychological effect. Moderate aerobic exercise such as running or swimming tends to be most effective. In addition, being tired may actually be caused, at least in part, by a lack of exercise—what the experts call "sedentary inertia" or "exercise deficiency"—in which case exercise is the best antidote.

316. Warm up before stretching. Stretching cold muscles can injure them. Warming up—by jogging in place for 5 to 10 minutes, for instance—prepares you for exercise by gradually increasing your heart rate and blood flow, raising the temperature of muscles, and improving muscle function. It may also decrease the chance of a sports injury.

317. Run away from diabetes. Doctors have long recommended exercise as a way to help control diabetes. And recent studies offer strong direct evidence that physical activity may actually help prevent Type 2 diabetes.

318. Work out in the garden. Use an old-fashioned lawn mower and you'll burn 420 to 480 calories an hour—as much as you would playing tennis. Spading, lifting, tilling, and raking can improve muscle tone and strength. Even the less strenuous forms of garden upkeep—weeding, trimming, raking—can burn about 300 calories an hour, if you work energetically at a constant pace.

319. To avoid overtraining and reduce the risk of injury, try cross training. Instead of running every day, alternate it with swimming—this will give your leg muscles and joints a needed rest between runs. And if you do hurt your knees or ankles while running, you won't have to stop exercising—you can keep on swimming to maintain your aerobic capacity.

320. Don't "run through" pain. If you feel pain (beyond mild discomfort) when exercising, stop. People often ignore pain or delay treating it, and thus aggravate the problem—so that full recovery can take weeks or months. The surest way to avoid such trouble is to treat any recurring ache or pain right away.

321. If you don't have time for long workouts, try 10-minute sessions. One study found that nine weekly 10-minute sessions offer the same cardiovascular benefits as three weekly 30-minute sessions. That's good news for beginning exercisers, who may find it easier to stick to shorter, more manageable workouts. Turn your coffee break into an exercise break. Try 10 minutes of brisk walking before work, 10 minutes of stair-climbing or a quick run at noon, and 10 minutes of rope jumping or cycling in the evening.

322. When shopping for new running shoes, take your old pair with you so that a knowledgeable salesperson can evaluate the wear pattern to help you choose a suitable shoe. Wear the socks you normally run in, and run around in the store after putting on the new shoes.

323. Before you buy an exercise shoe, try to bend it. The shoe should bend where the foot bends—at the ball; if it bends at mid-foot it will offer little support. It shouldn't bend too easily or be too stiff.

324. Exercise against aging. Regular exercise inhibits or even reverses many of the declines commonly associated with aging. A long-term regimen of three to five brisk 30-minute walks each week, for instance, may not only add years to your life, but also life to your years.

325. To prevent saddle soreness, use a gel-filled or sheepskin saddle or pad on your bike. The hard, narrow seats on racing bikes can be particularly uncomfortable for women, who tend to have more widely spaced "sit bones" than men. Special anatomically designed saddles are easy to install.

326. If you play golf, you can reap fitness rewards by walking instead of riding a cart. (Try to avoid courses where carts are required.) And if you carry your bag, you'll get an even more strenuous workout. Playing an 18-hole course you cover about five miles and burn an estimated 500 calories.

327. To get the most from a stair-climbing machine, don't lean on the rails or front monitor, since that reduces your energy expenditure. Hold the rails lightly—just enough to avoid losing your balance.

328. For a better walking workout on the treadmill, swing your arms. That way your movement is similar to cross-country skiing, one of the best calorie burners around. One study found that treadmill walkers, by adding vigorous arm motion, could boost their caloric expenditures by about 50%—from 10 calories per minute up to 15. This will also improve upper-body strength.

329. Walk hills to burn more calories. It's not surprising that you burn more calories when you walk uphill than on level ground. But, in fact, walking downhill also uses significantly more energy than walking on flat terrain.

330. Try not to run straight down a steep hill: instead, run down in a zigzag pattern, leaning slightly forward and keeping your knees bent. Or walk down it. Running downhill puts much more stress on joints and muscles in your feet and legs than running uphill. As you go down a hill, you speed up, your stride lengthens, and thus your impact with the ground increases. There's also an increased risk of muscle soreness the next day.

331. When exercising, use the "talk test" to make sure you aren't working out too strenuously. If you can just respond to conversation, your exercise intensity is just about right. If you can't talk, slow down. This test can be as accurate as heart rate monitors in gauging exercise intensity.

332. To reduce your risk of stroke, take a walk. A Yale University study of more than 9,000 white male veterans, aged 50 to 60, showed that those who reported inactive life styles were nearly seven times more likely to suffer a stroke than men who were moderately or very active. A daily walk of just one mile was found to be the minimum activity for reducing stroke risk.

333. Take the stairs. Several work-site studies have found that people who simply began using staircases (instead of elevators) improved their overall physical fitness by 10 to 15%. A person climbing stairs at the rate of two steps per second uses, on average, 18 calories per minute, or 360 calories in just 20 minutes.

334. If you play a sport and sometimes have low-back pain, try to correct muscle imbalances by becoming a little ambidextrous. Constantly rotating your lower back and hips in the same direction can produce recurrent muscle strain. So if you play golf, practice occasionally with an opposite-handed swing. In tennis warm-ups, try a few weaker-side forehand and backhand strokes. In baseball, try a few weaker-side pitches between batters.

335. Replace worn exercise shoes. They typically lose about one-third of their ability to absorb shock after 500 miles of use and may wear unevenly. Loss of cushioning in the shock-absorbent midsole occurs long before the outer sole or upper shoe shows wear.

336. Once the hot weather starts, build up your tolerance to outdoor exercise slowly. During the first week or two, your body will adjust by enlarging sweat glands and tiny blood vessels near the skin's surface.

337. Walk on sand or soft dirt to boost your energy expenditure by a third. It also exercises more of the muscles in the foot, especially if you walk barefoot.

338. To boost immunity, exercise regularly and moderately. Though long and intense exercise may actually depress immunity, moderate exercise may boost the body's ability to fight off colds and other illness.

339. Try cross-country skiing. In terms of all-around aerobic benefits, it's the front runner. Using muscles in the shoulders, back, chest, abdomen, buttocks, and legs, cross-country skiers can burn as many as 600 to 900 calories per hour. Cross-country skiing also spares your body the impact that running inflicts.

340. Drink, drink, drink. You can easily sweat away more than a quart of water during an hour of strenuous exercise, especially in hot weather. Dehydration can impair your performance, causing lethargy, nausea, and cramps, or even heat exhaustion. Drink even if you don't feel thirsty. For optimal hydration during strenuous endurance exercise, drink at least 16 to 20 ounces of fluid two hours before exercising and another 8 ounces 15 to 30 minutes before. While exercising, sip 4 to 6 ounces every 15 to 20 minutes.

341. After exercising, replace the fluid you've sweated off. Weigh yourself before and after your workout; drink one pint for each pound lost.

342. Make your own sports drink. For most exercisers, water is an ideal fluid replacement. But during a strenuous endurance event lasting more than an hour, slightly sugared beverages may help your body conserve its carbohydrate stores, maintain normal blood sugar levels, and thus delay fatigue. Special "sports drinks" supply the optimal amount of carbohydrates—4 to 8% concentration—for endurance exercise, plus small amounts of sodium and potassium. But, in fact, these drinks are nutritionally similar to diluted juice or soft drinks.

343. For the best sit-ups, keep your knees bent and your feet flat on the floor, and come up to no more than a 30° angle. Skip those old-fashioned straight-leg sit-ups; these can make you overarch and thus strain your lower back.

344. Exercise to help maintain a healthy blood pressure level. People with high blood pressure are generally advised to do aerobic exercise (such as cycling or brisk walking) and strength training with light weights. If you have high blood pressure, check with your doctor before beginning any exercise program. Be careful if you lift heavy weights or do isometric exercise—such as pushing against a wall or pressing palms together to build strength. Keep the intensity light to moderate, and rest between the brief bouts.

345. Try high-tech athletic socks, made of a variety of new synthetic materials, such as high-bulk Orlon (acrylic) and polypropylene. They are better at protecting your feet from friction, absorbing perspiration, and providing cushioning.

346. Here's a novel way to strengthen your forearm muscles, wrist, and grip, as well as increase flexibility. With one outstretched arm, hold a page of newspaper by a corner and crumble it up into a small ball as fast as you can using only that one hand. Repeat a few times, several times a week, as part of your regular exercise routine. This can help in a wide variety of sports, from tennis to rock climbing, as well as in daily activities.

347. When exercising outdoors on a cold day, don't overdress. Exercise raises body temperature significantly—even a moderate workout can make you feel that it's 30° warmer than it really is. So when you're about to run on a 25° day, dress for about 55°. In other words, dress so that you're slightly chilled when you first go out—once you start exercising, you'll warm up. And layer your clothing—that allows you to unzip and/or remove clothes in order to lower body temperature during strenuous exertion.

348. If you can't keep up your normal exercise routine, try to work out at least once a week to prevent "detraining." Studies show that exercising just one day a week can help people maintain their gains.

349. If your muscles are sore the day after strenuous exercise, the best remedy is to make those muscles work again by going back to the same exercise the next day, only less intensely.

350. Wear sunscreen when exercising in the sun. Many runners and other outdoor exercisers avoid sunscreens because they've heard that the creams can inhibit sweating and lead to overheating. But one study found that sunscreens might actually enhance heat dissipation slightly, which would be beneficial. Skin temperature rose less when people wore sunscreen than when they didn't. This may not be true of all products, so try different brands to see which works best for you when you exercise.

351. Always ice an acute injury immediately. Continue icing every 20 minutes during the next 48 hours. Applying heat can increase inflammation if done within the first day or two.

352. Take the following steps to relieve a stitch (a sharp pain in the side) that develops during exercise. Bend forward while tightening your abdomen. Breathe deeply and exhale slowly through pursed lips. Tighten your belt. If you aren't wearing one, push your fingers into the painful area. Also try stretching the abdominal muscles by raising your arms and reaching above your head.

353. When using a stationary bike or treadmill, set up a fan to blow directly on you as you exercise. The air blowing on your skin will cool you even faster than air-conditioning. A lack of air flow is one reason why a workout on an indoor cycle can be so much more tiring than the same amount of cycling outdoors, even in the hottest weather. The evaporation of sweat provides the most important cooling mechanism for your body—and this process is helped considerably if you have dry air flowing on your skin and around your body.

354. Always wear a helmet when cycling. Of the nation's 800 annual cycling deaths in the U.S., head injuries account for about 60%. If all cyclists wore helmets, perhaps half of these deaths and injuries could be avoided.

355. Wear your bike helmet right: tighten the straps so that the helmet can't tip forward or backward and so that you can open your mouth only a little. Don't wear the helmet tipped upward: it should sit level from front to back. If you can easily slip a finger between your head and the shell, the helmet is too big and you should consider buying a smaller one.

356. If you have osteoarthritis, the best thing you can do is exercise. Understandably, if you have joint pain you may have formed the habit of walking more slowly and doing as little as possible. If this is the case, you need to get moving again—slowly and gently, but definitely. It's a good idea to check with your physician first, and possibly get a referral to a physical therapist. You can also contact the Arthritis Foundation.

357. Use elastic bands if you want to become stronger but are intimidated by the idea of lifting dumbbells and barbells (and don't have access to weight machines). These long, wide bands provide the resistance you need to work your muscles. They are cheap, easy to carry around, and versatile. Available in sporting-goods stores, the bands often come with good illustrated booklets.

358. Add jumping rope to your workout to build cardiovascular endurance. It also helps improve coordination, speed, and agility. If you play a sport (such as tennis, basketball, or skiing) that requires bursts of speed and power, jumping rope can be particularly beneficial. It burns lots of calories: if you weigh 150 pounds and jump at 120 turns per minute, you'll burn about 12 calories a minute. And it's lower in impact and less hard on the knees than running, since you should jump only an inch or two off the ground.

359. Drink as much in the cold as in the heat. It's easy to become dehydrated when exercising in cold weather because of the water you lose from sweating and breathing (you have to warm and moisten the cold air you inhale). As you exhale you lose water; when you "see" your breath, you're seeing water droplets. Moreover, urine production is stimulated by the cold. Skip alcohol and caffeine; both dehydrate you. Alcohol gives you the illusion of warmth while it robs you of heat by dilating blood vessels near the skin's surface.

360. To boost your metabolic rate, exercise more. Your metabolic rate is the rate at which your body uses energy—the number of calories it burns in a given